Let's Talk

About

Sex

A biblical perspective on the subject of sex

Recognising the power of purity

Matthew Ashimolowo

© 2003 Matthew Ashimolowo

Published by Mattyson Media an imprint of MAMM
Matthew Ashimolowo Media Ministries

Visit our website: www.pastormatthew.com

ISBN 1 874646 59 7

Bible quotes are from the King James version Bible
unless otherwise stated.

Introduction

Ｔhe subject of this book is so touchy for Christians that it has become a rare topic on our bookstands. The views Christians hold on sexual matters have also made the world to see us as killjoys.

A generation is being raised in the Church that is sometimes under-informed from a biblical perspective because pulpiteers do not want to seize the moment and teach the subject on a Sunday morning. Where there is an absence of proper and correct information, people will turn to friends, movies, television, magazines, romance novels, music, peer groups or relatives.

The degree of a man's thirst determines how he behaves when he finds his water. Polluted water will not appeal to him if he has an alternative and his thirst can be controlled. But imagine a man in a desert who has not had water for about seven days. He finally finds an oasis where the water has just been troubled and the water looks reddish. Certainly the power of his thirst would overwhelm and becloud his judgement as to the dust contained in the water he drinks.

If our understanding of sex comes from everywhere else except God, the Church and the Bible, then our view will be lopsided and based on human ideas. Yet sometimes when the Church exercises that right to speak about sex, it only talks of sexual purity without making it clear that it involves more than being a virgin for the single person, and more than sexual fidelity to your spouse for the married.

It also is more than sexual abstinence for both the married and the single. It is a rounded matter that needs to be approached in a godly, yet informed way.

CHAPTER ONE

The Beauty of Sex

In the words of Dr Myles Munroe, "Unless purpose is known, abuse is inevitable." If you do not know the purpose of a thing you will use it abnormally. Of all the reasons for sex in Scripture, two stand out clearly.

The first is procreation...

And God blessed them, and God said unto them, Be fruitful, and multiply, and replenish the earth, and subdue it: and have dominion over the fish of the sea, and over the fowl of the air, and over every living thing that moveth upon the earth.
Genesis 1:28 (KJV)

The second is communication...

Let thy fountain be blessed: and rejoice with the wife of thy
youth. Let her be as the loving hind and pleasant roe; let her
breasts satisfy thee at all times; and be thou ravished always
with her love.
Proverbs 5:18-19 (KJV)

Several years ago I entered a general bookstore on a street corner in Africa. Young teens had just left school and stopped in
this bookstore probably to buy some of the things they needed
for their schoolwork. On the shelf was a book titled "God
Thought About Sex First." All the boys and girls giggled to
each other because the little they knew from what they had
either been told by friends or had been passed around, suddenly made sex to be a taboo subject for God to think about.

How can it be a taboo subject to God if He created this drive
in order to keep replenishing the earth and to communicate
love within marriage? How can it be a taboo to God if He pro-
nounced His blessing upon mankind?

So God created man in his own image, in the image of God
created he him; male and female created he them.
And God blessed them, and God said unto them, Be fruitful,
and multiply, and replenish the earth, and subdue it: and
have dominion over the fish of the sea, and over the fowl of
the air, and over every living thing that moveth upon the
earth.
Genesis 1:27-28 (KJV)

Rather we see from the onset that God's intention was for a

man and woman to live together as a couple before they engaged in sexual relationship. The initial and first couple in the Bible show us this.

> And Adam knew Eve his wife; and she conceived, and bare
> Cain, and said, I have gotten a man from the LORD.
> Genesis 4:1 (KJV)

Adam did not know his girlfriend. Eve was his wife from day one. Wrong teaching from the church has also given the impression that maybe sexual conjugation is a taboo subject. During the fourth century Saint Augustine, one of the early church leaders, made sex look like it must have been the forbidden fruit that God told Adam not to eat.

This possibly influenced the Catholic belief that priests should not marry. We who live today of course know the various consequences and abuse that have come out of such belief systems. The language the Bible uses conveys an expression of the fact that sex is designed for married couples.

> Flee fornication. Every sin that a man doeth is without the
> body; but he that committeth fornication sinneth against his
> own body.
> 1 Corinthians 6:18 (KJV)

> Meats for the belly, and the belly for meats: but God shall
> destroy both it and them. Now the body is not for
> fornication, but for the Lord; and the Lord for the body.
> 1 Corinthians 6:13 (KJV)

When it takes place outside of marriage, the Scripture clearly calls it a sin.

> Know ye not that the unrighteous shall not inherit the kingdom of God? Be not deceived: neither fornicators, nor idolaters, nor adulterers, nor effeminate, nor abusers of themselves with mankind, Nor thieves, nor covetous, nor drunkards, nor revilers, nor extortioners, shall inherit the kingdom of God.
> 1 Corinthians 6:9-10 (KJV)

In the passage just quoted, it makes reference to three key areas.

1. Fornicators - this is sexual intercourse participated in by a person who is not married.

2. Adulterers - these are people who are having sexual intercourse with a married person who is not their spouse. Or as the case may be if the married person has sex with single person, the married person in that act is an adulterer.

3. Effeminate and abusers of mankind - this is the third category and it refers to homosexuality and lesbianism.

God loves all humans; He loves homosexuals, but does not love or permit the act. Firstly, they are having sex outside the bounds of marriage; whether it is with the same sex or the opposite sex, the fact that it is outside of marriage, makes it unacceptable to God. Secondly the Bible does not make provision for two people of the same sex to be married. Thirdly people of the same sex cannot fulfil the purpose of sex, one of which is reproduction.

Later in this book we will see that for God, sexual conjugation is more like an act of worship and it is impossible for you to give acceptable worship in the wrong temple and in an unacceptable way.

Purity is not just an act, from the biblical perspective it is a lifestyle that Christians engage in.

And whatsoever ye do in word or deed, do all in the name of the Lord Jesus, giving thanks to God and the Father by him.
Colossians 3:17 (KJV)

This verse establishes that Christianity is not just a religion; it is what we do or say. It is a wholesome life. The question then comes, is it not hard to wait until you get married? Nothing good comes easy; those who wait for their spouse and wait until there is a solemnisation of their marriage can say: "I loved you before I knew you, to the extent that I kept myself for you."

CHAPTER TWO

The Defilement

ow can such a wonderful gift intended to bind two people together for life, intended as a medium of the highest communication between two people who have vowed to share the rest of their life, become so defiled? Time will not permit us to go as far back as antiquity to establish the fact that from the days of Hamurabi, of the great Babylonian kingdom, pornography and bizarre sexual practices have been around. But for us who live in these our times there was probably a greater paradigm shift in the Sixties, a period called, "The Times of the Sexual Revolution." Unfortunately, looking at the consequences of that revolution, it has become sexual exploitation.

> There is a way that seemeth right unto a man, but the end thereof are the ways of death.
> Proverbs 16:25 (KJV)

People fall into all forms of defilement, because of statements made to them, or things they conceive and desire to do. A man says to a lady, "You are gorgeous." But she does not take into account the fact that he may just want her for what she looks like; he does not love her for who she is. Or he says, "Look how happy we are." He did not mean to say, "I will be content with you alone." He is happy with her for the moment.

So people took what was a good idea from God and defiled it. Therefore today we have challenging situations. We have surrendered to our lusts and we have invited sexual thoughts into our minds and nurtured them to the point also where we have gone beyond nurturing them to deliberating and acting on them.

> Mortify therefore your members which are upon the earth;
> fornication, uncleanness, inordinate affection, evil
> concupiscence, and covetousness, which is idolatry:
> Colossians 3:5 (KJV)

The defilement of sex has been complicated also by the advent of television. This great communicator of several things is not the best communicator of love and sex. To learn about sex and love from television is like learning boxing from a defeated boxer. We must always remember that behind programmes we see on television, there are people who hold certain values. Their values are influencing the scripts they write and the programmes they choose to show us. And though censorship may have been introduced, in different parts of the world where censorship is enforced, certain images are not supposed to be shown until after nine in the evening. In some cases the reality is different.

How does sex outside marriage defile?

It simply marks down the person who is having it outside marriage. Sexual experience does not reinforce your ultimate value if it is not within marriage. If anything it marks you down as having been used and depreciated. When God called you a person of value, you have chosen to expose certain parts of your life with those with whom you might not have anything to do in the future.

> For thou hast possessed my reins: thou hast covered me in my mother's womb. I will praise thee; for I am fearfully and wonderfully made: marvellous are thy works; and that my soul knoweth right well.
> Psalm 139:13-14 (KJV)

Sex is defiled when we make it the basis on which we choose our spouses. The language today is "He or she has sex appeal." Ask anyone who has a happy home, and anyone who has had a disaster of a relationship or marriage and they will tell you that people who have the ability to communicate effectively and act in wisdom are better partners than how they perform in the bed.

If sex appeal brings a man to you, he is likely to abandon you if the going gets tough. Someone has said that eighty-five percent of men who impregnate a girl outside marriage end up leaving them or abandoning them.

> For as the heavens are higher than the earth, so are my ways higher than your ways, and my thoughts than your thoughts.
> Isaiah 55:9 (KJV)

A defilement of sex comes from the source from which a lot of people get their information. Young men sometimes get it from whom they hang around with; barber shops, peers, or once in a while when they have sneaked away and watched a certain movie or pornographic literature. And when people boast of their sexual prowess in barber shops, they never really tell us what part of the story is coloured, with the intention to impress us. Because the word out there among young men is that the greater your conquests, the greater your sexual prowess, the better your image among your 'homeboys.'

They never care how you use the girl, but certainly, when your story is out there that this one has 'laid' you and that one has 'laid' you, it hurts your reputation.

CHAPTER THREE

The Causes of Sexual Sin

In this chapter we will look at the following ten points.

1.   Flattery and flirtatious words

For the lips of a strange woman drop as an honeycomb, and
her mouth is smoother than oil:
Proverbs 5:3 (KJV)

To keep thee from the evil woman, from the flattery of the
tongue of a strange woman.
Proverbs 6:24 (KJV)

That they may keep thee from the strange woman, from the
stranger which flattereth with her words.
Proverbs 7:5 (KJV)

Imagine a bunch of young people singing "Your love is a 187, taking me to heaven." A lady visits the man she loves, or thinks she loves and before she knows it, he puts on a song that appeals to her senses, he makes the atmosphere right for his next move. Then he brings out what he knows a woman wants to hear. "Didn't they say a woman is from Venus and men are from Mars?" "Didn't they say a woman reacts to the appropriate words, and a man reacts to the appropriate action?" So he uses languages that solicit her trust. He says to her, "I can be trusted." That solicits privacy, and he says, "...and we can't tell anyone about us."

He uses language that shows he is being flirtatious and he is flattering her, "You're so smart, you're so sweet, you're very pretty, you're the best thing that ever happened to me." Every one of us at any one time wants information that builds our person, but also we like what builds our base person. Sometimes words will come that are really intended to bribe you. "I will buy you everything you want." Or, "I have met many girls, but none of them can stand your beauty." And if he is married and you remind him so, he says, "That woman at home, she doesn't understand that once in a while a man needs to play away games."

Foolishness is the only reason to allow yourself to be enticed by the empty words, promises or flattery you hear. But certainly these are one of the ways that people get to engage into sexual sin. Flirting and teasing are open invitations for trouble, it is better to say what you mean to this person and mean what you say. My mother used to say, "You do not stroke a cobra's head, because whether dead or alive, all cobras are deadly."

Flattery is further affirmed by all the images from Hollywood that give the impression that sex is more than it is. When a

The longer you are where you should not be, the quicker you are likely to do the things you should not do. We have therefore raised a generation who seem to think they know everything about sex but unfortunately they have turned out to be damaged, because they have been left with images and consequences beyond what they can possibly think or handle.

There are some of us today who are struggling with certain issues that did not quite start with us, but are products of the sexual indiscipline of our forbearers.

6.   Hanging around wrong places

Passing through the street near her corner; and he went the
way to her house, In the twilight, in the evening, in the black
and dark night:
Proverbs 7:8-9 (KJV)

One of satan's strategies is to make you fall into the trick that a person you have met has such great and intense love for you, so great that you should cross the boundaries drawn by the Word of God. The impact of course is dire, and when you want to stop, something from the realm of the flesh says, like the Nike advert, "Just do it!" Feelings are very tricky, the line between love and infatuation is very slim, and the more physical you become with a person, the more your judgement becomes clouded. The closer you think you are, the further away you are from being able to keep the person.

But every man is tempted, when he is drawn away of his
own lust, and enticed. Then when lust hath conceived, it
bringeth forth sin: and sin, when it is finished, bringeth forth
death.
James 1:14-15 (KJV)

We do not only hang around the wrong places with people whom we go with. Sometimes people go to seek sexual satisfaction with prostitutes or pick up men or women from bars and clubs. They think in the words of Miss Turner, "What's love go to do with it? It's just sexual union." Unfortunately from a biblical perspective, the truth is you may attempt to do that but you cannot get full satisfaction without the other unions which are meant to be there; spiritual union, emotional union, true oneness. As a matter of fact, if you lie down with dogs you will come up with what they have.

> For without are dogs, and sorcerers, and whoremongers, and murderers, and idolaters, and whosoever loveth and maketh a lie.
> Revelation 22:15 (KJV)

> Don't you realize that your bodies are actually parts and members of Christ? So should I take part of Christ and join him to a prostitute? Never!
> 1 Corinthians 6:15 (Living)

It is interesting that some men will describe themselves today as dogs, so if somebody let the dogs out, put the dogs back in their kennel. If you go and pick a person to meet your sexual conjugation, or you pick a person who is promiscuous and they are not committed to Christ and therefore bringing discipline to that aspect of their life, it is foolhardy to think that a person who had a variety of sexual partners will turn around to be faithful, and that one day they will suddenly turn around and be single minded in their love towards you.

> As a dog returneth to his vomit, so a fool returneth to his folly.
> Proverbs 26:11 (KJV)

It is only God that can bring a transformation that will make the person walk in marital fidelity. True love waits, and for a single person a relationship is too serious if you begin to get into the territories reserved for married people.

> My little children, let us not love in word, neither in tongue; but in deed and in truth.
> 1 John 3:18 (KJV)

7.   Suggestive clothing and slyness

> And, behold, there met him a woman with the attire of an harlot, and subtil of heart.
> Proverbs 7:10 (KJV)

It does not take a rocket scientist to know that people who have an intention to convey a message of sexiness design much of today's clothing. That probably informs why they say someone is "dressed to kill." They call that kind of clothes the "Come and get me" way of dressing. The argument is two-way. One view would say, "Why shouldn't a person wear what they like, it makes them feel comfortable and proud of themselves?"

The Scripture does talk of the lust of the eyes.

> For all that is in the world, the lust of the flesh, and the lust of the eyes, and the pride of life, is not of the Father, but is of the world.
> 1 John 2:16 (KJV)

No matter how anointed a person is, what you look at is what you meditate on. What you meditate on is what you speak about. We wear these clothes so we will be attractive, but really true attractiveness is not based on the scantiness of your clothes, but the beauty that exudes from within. However, such clothing has dragged someone into a problem.

8. Bad company and sexual indiscipline

And, behold, there met him a woman with the attire of an harlot, and subtil of heart.
(She is loud and stubborn; her feet abide not in her house:
Proverbs 7:10-11 (KJV)

Abstain from all appearance of evil.
1 Thessalonians 5:22 (KJV)

Ye adulterers and adulteresses, know ye not that the friendship of the world is enmity with God? whosoever therefore will be a friend of the world is the enemy of God.
James 4:4 (KJV)

We are essentially social beings, we cannot perform by ourselves for too long or we begin to degenerate. We need the company of other people. But if we are being influenced by ungodly friends to the point where we question the voracity and authenticity of our faith, then there is a problem. It is not only the company, but also the sexual indiscipline practiced innocently in the beginning sometimes, heavy petting, fondling, innocent little games, before it becomes a major problem. There is a difference between a holy hug and a continuous back massage. That is the reason why Paul warns us, "It is better not to touch a woman."

Now concerning the things whereof ye wrote unto me: It is good for a man not to touch a woman.
1 Corinthians 7:1 (KJV)

This man of God must be saying, "Don't start what you cannot stop." The statistics of your body, the human skin is eighteen square inches. It is one sixteenth of an inch in thickness, it weighs eight pounds. There are five million nerve endings all over our body that are connected to our skin. Whenever our body is touched, those nerve endings serve like electronic cables that take messages to the brain. These nerve endings are seventy-two feet in all, carrying fifteen feet of blood vessels. The moment your body is touched the message goes from your internal nerves that are connected to your skin, through to your spinal cord and from your spinal cord, the nerves carry it to your brain. Your brain counts the feelings, your brain stores the feelings, and your brain can retrieve previously stores touches and feelings. You can be imprinted by a touch; you can sit and remember Joe's touch and Janet's kiss because your brain has stored in it a hard disk from which it can be retrieved.

When men go for relationships they often want sex. For a lot of girls who ended up pregnant or broken, all they wanted was a touch. Something they could also call up and remember, but it went beyond a touch. Fornication is more than just the act of sexual penetration; it involves all sexual sins performed outside of marriage. The word fornication comes from the Greek *pornea,* which means *all forms of sexual misconduct.* You must avoid the mistake of thinking that making love will make a person love you.

We must not be sexually promiscuous - they paid for that, remember, with twenty-three thousand deaths in one day!
1 Corinthians 10:8 (Message)

9.   Lack of sobriety or propriety

*I have peace offerings with me; this day have I payed my
vows. Therefore came I forth to meet thee, diligently to seek
thy face, and I have found thee.*
Proverbs 7:14-15 (KJV)

One of the things a person should aim to develop immediately
upon being born again is a renewed mind.

*I beseech you therefore, brethren, by the mercies of God, that
ye present your bodies a living sacrifice, holy, acceptable unto
God, which is your reasonable service.
And be not conformed to this world: but be ye transformed
by the renewing of your mind, that ye may prove what is that
good, and acceptable, and perfect, will of God.*
Romans 12:1-2 (KJV)

*Therefore if any man be in Christ, he is a new creature: old
things are passed away; behold, all things are become new.*
2 Corinthians 5:17 (KJV)

I am an advocate of not allowing people to serve immediately
after they get born again. They should spend at least six
months to a year trying to clean their hard disk of old ways and
lifestyle and beginning to develop new qualities, commitment
and view points as believers.

Following salvation, part of the renewal of the mind should be
to learn Christian disciplines; worship, prayer, Bible study,
witnessing, relating to the household of faith, stewardship of
giving, and serving, before attempting to go into matters of
relationships.

10. Unfaithfulness

For the goodman is not at home, he is gone a long journey:
He hath taken a bag of money with him, and will come home
at the day appointed.
Proverbs 7:19-20 (KJV)

This passage says a man should run from a promiscuous
woman, because she would burn him, whether home or away.
And for the lady she should not play house; cooking a man's
food, running his errand when he is not your husband.

A person who is unfaithful will make a poor husband.
Experience has shown that people who get drunk, do drugs and
fool around make poor partners.

He that walketh with wise men shall be wise: but a
companion of fools shall be destroyed.
Proverbs 13:20 (KJV)

It is important to know where men and women must stop.
Whenever they want to go to boundaries or territories which
they call love and it does not fit into that description, you must
clearly let them know.

Prince Absalom, David's son, had a beautiful sister named
Tamar. And Prince Amnon (her half brother) fell desperately
in love with her.... But as she was standing there before him,
he grabbed her and demanded, "Come to bed with me, my
darling." "Oh, Amnon," she cried. "Don't be foolish! Don't
do this to me! You know what a serious crime it is in Israel.
But he wouldn't listen to her; and since he was stronger than
she, he forced her. Then suddenly his love turned to ha

and now he hated her more than he had loved her. "Get out
of here!" he snarled at her.

2 Samuel 13:1, 11-12, 14-15 (Living)

CHAPTER FOUR

The Consequences of Sexual Sin

When HIV/Aids took the world by storm, people came to an awareness of what effect unprotected sex could have. However, apart from diseases, we are not given the impression that there is any consequence to sex outside of marriage.

From our study of the book of Proverbs we can establish that it leads to:

1.   Bitterness

Every attraction you allow to become a distraction will provoke ungodly actions that will leave your salvation in fractions. To be attracted to people is very natural, but to act on every attraction will lead to grievous dangers. The degree of your bitterness when the relationship is over will be determined by how much investment you made in the relationship before it was over.

2.   Pain

> Her feet go down to death; her steps take hold on hell.
> Proverbs 5:5 (KJV)

This passage describes the sensual woman who only leads to the path of pain and hurt, and although the passage talks of a woman it could also refer to a man. God never condemns a person for having a desire, but acting on your desire in an illicit way will put you in danger of hell fire. Those who act on every craving of their appetite put themselves in grave danger. If you wait for your hunger to subside, you will enjoy the meal at the appropriate time, otherwise the pain you bring upon yourself and the children that might follow is almost indescribable. However, when seasons and times of emotional madness arise, no one remembers or considers the pain and consequence of sexual sin.

The passage says that her house leads to hell. So to walk away from the counsel of God is to expose oneself to a hellish life on earth and a possible one in eternity.

3.   Weak willed

Once the guard is let down, there seems to be a path of least resistance that one walks.

> Lest thou shouldest ponder the path of life, her ways are
> moveable, that thou canst not know them.
> Proverbs 5:6 (KJV)

The weak willed man who has a woman visiting, often misinterprets affections of a woman to mean a desire for sex. When a woman touches a man the message he gets is, it is no longer time to play games, it is action time.

Strong will on the other hand is not the answer. It is learning to be led and controlled by the Holy Spirit that matters the most.

> For as many as are led by the Spirit of God, they are the sons of God.
> Romans 8:14 (KJV)

The reason is because when you became born-again your hormones were not replaced with a Christian hormone; you must still keep yourself pure, keep yourself in check or else you will go the path many have gone previously. Giving in to sexual pressure and when you do give in, you lose out later. When you do not give in, you win later.

4.   Wasted Life

> Lest thou give thine honour unto others, and thy years unto the cruel:
> Proverbs 5:9 (KJV)

Hollywood will not paint for us the various consequences of sexual sin. It will not include for us the reality of broken homes, broken hearts, unplanned pregnancy, abortion, and the chances of the family living on welfare, a lower quality of life, sexually transmitted diseases, HIV and Aids.

Today we see right before our eyes the devastating effect of sexually transmitted diseases and its rampant increase particularly among teenagers. The level of the HIV/Aids problem in South Africa for example is forty-five per cent and people are now talking about a possible HIV genocide in that part of the world. The irony of getting HIV is that sometimes people look nice and young and therefore we think they could not be carriers.

5.   Financial Ruin

Lest strangers be filled with thy wealth; and thy labours be in the house of a stranger;
Proverbs 5:10 (KJV)

It is interesting that people try to buy love. If you are trying to buy someone's love it will not take long before you realise that not only would you lose your body, you would lose your money. When we look again at the verse just quoted, it seems to say that before you take off your clothes, you need to count the cost. Are you willing to pay the price for what you are about to do? Because if nobody else mentions the consequence of sexual sin, you have to understand that the wages of sin is still death. Who said pre-marital sex is free? Someone always pays one way or another.

6.   Bad Reputation

I was almost in all evil in the midst of the congregation and assembly.
Proverbs 5:14 (KJV)

Imagine the Christian who succumbs to the pressure of the moment, the madness of the season and goes beyond the call of duty and even tries to sleep with one they do not know. The people you know themselves are a problem, how much more exposing them and releasing yourself into a sexual relationship with a person whom you do not share fidelity and commitment in marriage.
To have sex with strangers is like handing over your bank

account to people you have never known to draw as much as they want. A man may look prim and proper, but you may fail to realise that the same Doctor Jekyll can turn again and be Mister Hyde.

7.   Trapped

His own iniquities shall take the wicked himself, and he shall
be holden with the cords of his sins.
Proverbs 5:22 (KJV)

There are some boundaries that are better not crossed because once they are crossed, it is hard to shake them off. The people with whom you sleep with leave something with you and you leave something with them. If a man has uncleanness, he brings it to you.

8.   Increased perversity

He shall die without instruction; and in the greatness of his
folly he shall go astray.
Proverbs 5:23 (KJV)

Once you desire to be stimulated, you never want it to stop. One degree of stimulation provokes another level; it is what I call the Pringles experience. My son once bought the crisps called Pringles. I had seen the advert on the television that once you eat it you do not want to stop. I am not into crisps, but on this occasion when my son bought it, I tried one, I reached for the second, the third, and the fourth and went on and on and almost finished his pack of Pringles before he came back from the kitchen.

Once you start the stimulation, you want to go to the penetration. So do not start a fire you do not know how to quench. If you want to be special for the person with whom you will share the future, do not unwrap your Christmas gift before Christmas. Do not unwrap with every date you go out on, or you will soon be out before your sell by date.

9. Poverty

For by means of a whorish woman a man is brought to a piece of bread: and the adulteress will hunt for the precious life.
Proverbs 6:26 (KJV)

10. Ruination

But whoso committeth adultery with a woman lacketh understanding: he that doeth it destroyeth his own soul.
Proverbs 6:32 (KJV)

11. Foolishness

But whoso committeth adultery with a woman lacketh understanding: he that doeth it destroyeth his own soul.
Proverbs 6:32 (KJV)

The sweet mouth of a promiscuous woman must not become the trap a young man falls into and forgets his calling, his gift and salvation, and because your friends say it is okay it does not mean it is. Those who allow their friends to dictate what they do are taking their direction from a man who himself he is lost.

12. Dishonour

> A wound and dishonour shall he get; and his reproach shall
> not be wiped away.
> Proverbs 6:33 (KJV)

13. Hurt

> A wound and dishonour shall he get; and his reproach shall
> not be wiped away.
> Proverbs 6:33 (KJV)

Men and women act differently towards sexual relationships. It may hurt a man that the relationship is over, but because most men go into sex with their physical body, once it is over they have forgotten. Women are different, a woman keeps the memory of what she has experienced, because in most cases a woman goes into it spirit, soul and body. For some men the commitment is only as long as the act. So if a woman thinks such a person loves her automatically and therefore has a commitment with her she has made a mistake.

There are too many consequences to be enumerated in this passage.

Unwanted pregnancy, abortion, heartbreak, a bad memory, physical ill health and a loss of respect.

Imagine the fact that when men want to describe what they have done to a woman, if she is not their wife they say, "They socked it to her." "They misused her." "They did her." "They slew her." When the Scripture will talk of sexual copulation for the unmarried it will say, "And he laid with her." For those who are married it will say, "He knew his wife." There is a sense of intimacy in the case of husband and wife. No wonder young men will say of girls they have slept with, "She is an easy lay or she is a hard lay." Many guys have 'laid' with loads of women who are not their wives.

CHAPTER FIVE

The Tabernacle (a type and a shadow)

Know ye not that ye are the temple of God, and that the
Spirit of God dwelleth in you?
If any man defile the temple of God, him shall God destroy;
for the temple of God is holy, which temple ye are.
1 Corinthians 3:16-17 (KJV)

Following the fall of man in the Garden of Eden, his subsequent actions have been to devalue, degenerate and belittle what God hallows or holds in high esteem. Sexual intimacy is the highest form of intimacy among mortals. It is probably the deepest, strongest, hunger we express aside from eating food. When it takes place between two people, who share a covenant of marriage, there is a level of intimacy that is almost inexplicable. That is why if it is messed up; one's sense of understanding of intimacy with God gets messed up. In other words if your sexuality is messed up, your worship will be messed up, and if your love life is out of order, your devotion will also be.

A woman's body is like the tabernacle in the Old Testament. The Old Testament tabernacle had three parts; an outer court, a holy place or an inner court and the holy of holies. The outer court stands for the flesh, the body. The inner court stands for the soul, while the holy of holies stands for the spirit.

In the outer court was the altar of sacrifice for sin and a laver or a basin that also served more as a reflective glass, so that when you washed you also could see if you were clean or not. Before you even approach the laver for washing, you must have placed your sacrifice on the altar. In the same vein also, one of the things that touches a woman's heart is the ability to know and to bring gifts and to show value.

The laver is supposed to be a place of washing. If a man is unclean in his heart, if he does not come to the laver, it stops his fellowship with God. Likewise a man also who is in adultery or uncleanness. It stops the intimacy between him and his wife. Women can sometimes tell when their husbands who are sleeping with them are really not there with them, but with somebody else.

When the cleansing is done and the fellowship is established the second part of the tabernacle is the holy place. In the holy place there is a lamp stand, a table of shewbread, a veil that divides the holy place from the holy of holies. There is also the altar of incense.

The lamp stand obviously stands for the fact that the man should illuminate the woman's mind, be a priest and a challenger of her faith. He should bring her into revelation and truth by stroking her mind. A man who is able to stroke a woman's mind will bring her into greater blessings.

The table of shewbread is a place where friendship is established. Bread was never to be lacking on that table, just as the bond of friendship was never to be lacking between two people in spite of the years of marriage.

The altar of incense is where incense was burnt to God continuously. Symbolically it stands for sweet friendship, sweet relationship and that which touches the other person and causes them to respond also in love.

Between the holy place and the holy of holies is a veil. Only one man was permitted by God to push aside the veil and go into the holy of holies. For a woman who has not known a man, there is a little skin that covers the vagina known as the hymen. Just as the high priest was supposed to be the only one to go past the hymen into the holy of holies, God's intention was that there should be only one man in a woman's life. It is interesting to realise that at a point when a man is aroused, the male organ experiences erection through the rush of blood into it, to prepare it to fulfil a blood covenant.

On the day of the first copulation with a woman who is a virgin and the hymen is broken, the blood of the woman rests on the man, and covenant is established. This makes it a symbol of worship. Imagine a role reversal if God were to turn the type and shadow of the tabernacle into the real thing. Imagine the scenario where the high priest was to enter the holy of holies and he was unprepared, unclean or he was not the right person. In the Old Testament the high priest would die if he were unclean or not the right person. Imagine if people who go into having sexual relationships with other people who are not their spouses and such happens.

Therefore, as far as scripture is concerned, sexual relationship is not just lovemaking. It is covenant worship between two people who have vowed to share their lives. Not worship as in veneration, but worship as in 'worth-ship'. Recognising the worth of one another. So many have been 'laid' but not loved.
In sexual relationships the male organ is the altar. That is why

God, even in speaking to the Jews said that is where they have to circumcise as a symbol of surrender to Him.

> And ye shall circumcise the flesh of your foreskin; and it
> shall be a token of the covenant betwixt me and you.
> And he that is eight days old shall be circumcised among
> you, every man child in your generations, he that is born in
> the house, or bought with money of any stranger, which is
> not of thy seed.
> Genesis 17:11-12 (KJV)

What are altars for?

They certainly are for worship, but the altar can be altered. If you go everywhere and release yourself, you have altered your altar, you have desecrated your altar, and you have violated your purity. Sexual purity therefore is not just because God wants you to keep yourself and not have sex until marriage but because it is a form of worship and it is a symbol of your dedication that you have kept your body, which is His temple. When you have sex with a person who is not your spouse, if you enter them, or they enter you, you will get what they have. You become one with what you lay down with.

Have you observed how that in marriage, women drop their name and take the name of the man? That is one of the highest symbols of covenant. It is the taking on of the man's destiny. When Reuben slept with his father's wife, his father said, he shall be unstable as the waters. In other words it was to say he would lose control. And to lose control of your emotion and desires makes you unworthy of possessing your possession. No wonder the power of the covenant of Israel passed down rather to Joseph and not to Reuben the firstborn.

The same thing applies to the man who says, "But we are

engaged, our families know each other, we're looking forward to the day of marriage." When you have sex while waiting to marry you curse the foundation of your marriage, you prepare yourself for divorce and separation.

CHAPTER SIX

The Deliverance

Y ou must recognise the fact that it takes extra strength and commitment to go against a popular flow.

For the grace of God that bringeth salvation hath appeared to all men, Teaching us that, denying ungodliness and worldly lusts, we should live soberly, righteously, and godly, in this present world;
Titus 2:11-12 (KJV)

We live at a time when people see you as a deviant for choosing sexual purity and teaching that sex is only for marriage. However, even those who promoted free sex in the fifties, sixties and seventies are now beginning to say they wish they could turn the clock around. The extra mile includes of course understanding the fact that society essentially has put man on the moon, but does not have an intention to help people live differently or live according to the Word of God. You must have an understanding that society is prepared to spend so much money to teach you on how to drive a car, but not how to run a home.

In a well-furnished kitchen there are not only crystal goblets and silver platters, but waste cans and compost buckets - some containers used to serve fine meals, others to take out the garbage.
2 Timothy 2:20 (Message)

Run away from infantile indulgence. Run after mature righteousness - faith, love, peace - joining those who are in honest and serious prayer before God.
2 Timothy 2:22 (Message)

If you are in a relationship, refusal to give in to sexual involvement outside of marriage is a way of telling the other person that you are worth more than a thrill and more than a momentary gratification. But that you are a well prepared meal worth waiting for. To find your deliverance you must understand that easy sex or cheap sex does not make you more romantic. Practicing before your marriage does not make you prepared, you are more like a man practicing medicine before he got to medical school, because he wants to be a good doctor. It is better to wait for the appropriate seasons.

A garden inclosed is my sister, my spouse; a spring shut up, a fountain sealed.... Awake, O north wind; and come, thou south; blow upon my garden, that the spices thereof may flow out. Let my beloved come into his garden, and eat his pleasant fruits.
Song of Songs 4:12,16 (KJV)
We seem to have a world of reversals today. Certain parts of

Let's Talk About Sex

the body have always been called 'private parts' and I think we need to keep private parts private. We need to go back to the original definition of what private means. It means it is only accessible to the persons with whom you become one flesh.

> But strong meat belongeth to them that are of full age, even those who by reason of use have their senses exercised to discern both good and evil.
> Hebrews 5:14 (KJV)

A cure for sexual sin

1. Faithfulness

> Drink waters out of thine own cistern, and running waters out of thine own well. Let thy fountains be dispersed abroad, and rivers of waters in the streets. Let them be only thine own, and not strangers' with thee. Let thy fountain be blessed: and rejoice with the wife of thy youth.
> Let her be as the loving hind and pleasant roe; let her breasts satisfy thee at all times; and be thou ravished always with her love.
> Proverbs 5:15-19 (KJV)

It is interesting to note that even unsaved men prefer ladies from churches, because while the men may have philandered around, yet they want marital fidelity. Within marriage sex carries no condemnation, but outside of it, it is all condemnation and guilt.

God says such as practice immorality will not enter His kingdom and He has not changed His mind on it.

Now the works of the flesh are manifest, which are these;

59

Adultery, fornication, uncleanness, lasciviousness,
Idolatry, witchcraft, hatred, variance, emulations, wrath,
strife, seditions, heresies, Envyings, murders, drunkenness,
revellings, and such like: of the which I tell you before, as I
have also told you in time past, that they which do such
things shall not inherit the kingdom of God.
Galatians 5:19-21 (KJV)

2. Define the boundaries

Where you stand on sexual matters needs to be known as soon
as you meet a man. Vague statements like, "Oh I believe in
keeping ourselves sexually pure," are not enough. You must
affirm the fact that he keeps himself sexually pure and so
should the woman affirm this to the man before the relationship continues. You can be so quick to show your body, you
should not put on display what is not for sale.

I hate them with perfect hatred: I count them mine enemies.
Psalm 139:22 (KJV)

3. Run

God will not stop you if you remove your trousers, neither will
He stop you from jumping into the bed. The Holy Spirit will
not resist your hand when you begin "Body ministry" with the
other person. It is your responsibility to flee fornication.

Flee fornication. Every sin that a man doeth is without the
body; but he that committeth fornication sinneth against his
own body.
1 Corinthians 6:18 (KJV)
Ask anyone, the spur of the moment decisions are often dan-

gerous. For a man as soon as his body is touched within three seconds, hormones are released by his brain that cause him to make decisions based on his emotions and not his thought faculty. For the woman it is within twenty seconds.

Flee fornication. Every sin that a man doeth is without the body; but he that committeth fornication sinneth against his own body.
1 Corinthians 6:18 (KJV)

But thou, O man of God, flee these things; and follow after righteousness, godliness, faith, love, patience, meekness.
1 Timothy 6:11 (KJV)

4. Know the Word

The knowledge of the Word helps you in your discernment. The knowledge of the Word builds boundaries around your life. The knowledge of the Word helps you to decide how far you want to go. It is only the Word of God that teaches sexual purity, not any of today's literature outside of Christianity, and therefore you need to know the Word. Take time to study God's Word, particularly as it relates to the subject of sexual purity.

5. Take a vow of purity

I made a covenant with mine eyes; why then should I think upon a maid?
Job 31:1 (KJV)

A man must know his limit and therefore stay within it. To go beyond your limit is like walking into the zone of temptation without the leading of God, the consequence could be devastating. Do not set your mind on sexual sin. The Bible teaches us to meditate on that which is pure and acceptable.

> Finally, brethren, whatsoever things are true, whatsoever
> things are honest, whatsoever things are just, whatsoever
> things are pure, whatsoever things are lovely, whatsoever
> things are of good report; if there be any virtue, and if there
> be any praise, think on these things.
> Philippians 4:8 (KJV)

Seek and pray consistently for the grace of God and His ability to walk in purity. Recognise the fact that sex is a spiritual issue and you cannot separate your worship of God on Sunday and what you do with your body on Monday. Therefore sexual purity and spiritual purity are interwoven. Have you fallen into sexual sin before? Repent, reclaim your confidence and forgiveness in God and now walk and maintain sexual integrity. Where there has been sexual sin and a need to find cleansing, there must first be exposure of the sin to God. Disclosure of its impact on your life to God and find enclosure through His power.

In effect, God sees sex as a beautiful thing reserved for those who have paid the price of waiting and have shared the covenant of marriage and therefore have the rights of fulfilling their relationship through consummation.

Covenant

A promise of purity

Lord, realising that my body is Yours and that You live in me, I ask you this day for Your help to keep myself sexually pure until marriage. I promise to keep this covenant and to resist any temptation to break it. I ask that You will also keep my mate-to-be. Keep them in Your love and protect them from all danger.

In Your perfect time, bring us together in such a way that we will know for sure that we were meant for one another.

Lord, You always keep Your promise. Help me to keep mine.

"Know therefore that the Lord thy God, He is God, the faithful God, which keepeth covenant and mercy with them that love Him and keep His commandments to a thousand generations."
Deuteronomy 7:9

Signature _____

Date _____